CONTENTS

PASTEST REVISION BOOKS FOR MRCP 1

PasTest publish a wide range of revision books including:

MCQs in Basic Medical Sciences for MRCP 1
300 exam-based MCQs with answers and detailed explanatory notes

MRCP 1 Practice Exams: 2nd edition
Five complete MCQ Papers (300 MCQs) covering favourite Royal College topics

MRCP 1 MCQ Revision Book: 3rd edition
300 MCQs arranged by subject with correct answers and teaching notes, plus one complete mock exam

MRCP 1 Past Topics: A Revision Syllabus: 2nd edition
Contains authoritative lists of past topics which have occurred in the Royal College examination over the past 5 years

Explanations to the RCP Past Papers
Correct answers and teaching notes related to the Royal College Green and Blue books of actual past exam questions

MRCP Part 1 MCQs with Key Topic Summaries: 2nd edition
200 MCQs related to current examination syllabus with 200 comprehensive topic summaries

Membership at your Fingertips: MCQs on Disk
The disk contains 650 MCQs. Clear and concise teaching notes with every question

Oxford Textbook of Medicine MCQs: 3rd edition
375 new MCQs related to the 1995 Oxford Textbook of Medicine and ideal for subject based revision

For full details of all our revision books contact PasTest today on **01565 755226** for a free copy of our current book catalogue and price list. Books sent by return of post worldwide.

For full details contact:

PasTest, Egerton Court, Parkgate Estate,
Knutsford, Cheshire WA16 8DX
Telephone 01565 755226 Fax 01565 650264

INTRODUCTION

PasTest's MRCP Part 1 Pocket Books are designed to help the busy examination candidate to make the most of every opportunity to revise. With this little book in your pocket, it is the work of a moment to open it, choose a question, decide upon your answers and then check the answer on the back of the page. Revising "on the run" in this manner is both reassuring (if your answer is correct) and stimulating (if you find any gaps in your knowledge).

Each book contains 100 exam-based MCQs arranged by subject. Each author is a subject specialist who has based his selection of questions on past Royal College papers, and questions have also been designed specifically to address the basic sciences topics which have increasing prominence in the examination.

Each question consists of an initial statement followed by five possible completions, ABCDE. There is no restriction on the number of true or false items in a question. It is possible for all items in a question to be true or for all to be false. The four most important points of technique are:

1. Read the question carefully and be sure you understand it.
2. Mark your response clearly, correctly and accurately.
3. Use reasoning to work out your answer, but if you do not know the answer and cannot work it out, indicate "don't know".
4. The best possible way to obtain a good mark is to have as wide a knowledge as possible of the topics being tested in the examination.

It is possible to improve your mark by educated guessing, but this must be done with great care as incorrect answers are given a mark of –1 in the exam. You can use the books in this series to work out whether or not you are a good guesser by making a special mark against the responses that you have guessed before you check whether your responses are correct.

To get the best value from this book you should commit yourself to an answer for each item before you check the correct answer. With the answers on the back of each page, it can be tempting to find out which answers are correct before you have really decided on your own answer. But it is only by being sure of your own responses that you can ascertain which questions you would find difficult in the examination. Use the check boxes to mark your answers, or mark the parts of a question that you found difficult so that next time you look at the question you will be able to home in on your own personal areas of difficulty.

Books like the ones in this series, which consist of MCQs in subject categories, can help you to home in on specific topics and to isolate your weaknesses. You should plan a revision timetable to help you spread your time fairly over the range of subjects likely to appear in the examination. PasTest's *MRCP Part 1 Past Topics: A Revision Syllabus* will help you to work out which subjects deserve most of your revision time.

An effective revision plan should also include opportunities to practice your exam technique. Books of MCQ Practice Exams are indispensable and you should make time to sit at least two or three complete practice papers under timed conditions before the day of the actual examination arrives.

PasTest Revision Courses for MRCP 1

For 25 years PasTest, the leading independent specialists in post-graduate medical education, have been delivering top quality courses which have helped many thousands of doctors to pass the demanding MRCP Part 1 examination.

Our six-day MRCP Part 1 revision courses run three times each year at a convenient central London venue. Each delegate receives detailed course notes consisting of approximately 250 pages of exam-based MCQs with answers and comprehensive notes, plus many explanatory handouts.

✓ Learn from experienced and talented tutors with up-to-date knowledge of the requirements of the exam

✓ Teaching sessions focus on "favourite" exam topics and highlight possible areas of difficulty

✓ Four full practice exams enable you to constantly monitor your performance as the course progresses

For full details of the range of PasTest books and courses available for MRCP Part 1 candidates, contact PasTest today:

PasTest, Egerton Court, Parkgate Estate,
Knutsford, Cheshire WA16 8DX
Telephone: 01565 755226 Fax: 01565 650264

RHEUMATOLOGY

Mark your answers with a tick (True) or a cross (False) in the box provided. Leave the box blank for 'Don't know'.

1. The following are recognised features of rheumatoid arthritis:

☐ A ankle oedema

☐ B iritis

☐ C mouth ulcers

☐ D upper motor neurone signs

☐ E splenomegaly

2. In the treatment of rheumatoid arthritis

☐ A indomethacin is the safest NSAID when used in conventional doses

☐ B the proteinuria caused by gold is irreversible

☐ C patients on D-penicillamine need regular ophthalmic examination

☐ D methotrexate can cause a life-threatening pneumonitis

☐ E trimethoprim increases the antifolate effect of methotrexate

3. Activation of complement

☐ A cannot occur without the participation of immunoglobulins

☐ B results in increased capillary permeability

☐ C protects cells from lysis by stabilising cell membranes

☐ D does not occur in serum heated to 56c for 30 minutes

☐ E leads to the migration of neutrophils into sites of inflammation

Answers overleaf

1. A C D E

Ankle oedema may be a feature of cardiac failure, constrictive pericarditis or amyloid and nephrotic syndrome. Mouth ulcers may be associated with sicca syndrome, drugs or neutropenia. Splenomegaly is a feature of Felty's syndrome. Cervical cord compression may occur with subluxation leading to upper motor neurone neuropathy; mononeuritis multiplex and peripheral nerve entrapment are also common. Iritis is no more common than in the general population.

2. D E

Recent literature suggests azapropazone to have the highest and ibuprofen the lowest risk of adverse events. Gold produces a rash, leucopenia and thrombocytopenia; proteinuria tends to be reversible on stopping the drug. D-penicillamine has an association with myasthenic syndrome; hydroxychloroquine requires ophthalmic review. Methotrexate is an antifolate drug and its effect is increased by other antifolates, except sulphasalazine. Methotrexate can cause a pneumonitis and hepatitis. Cyclosporin A may also be therapeutic; it inhibits the production of interleukin 2 (IL-2) by activated T-cells and reduces IL-2 receptor expression.

3. B D E

Complement activation by the 'alternative pathway' occurs in the absence of antibodies by hydrolysis of C3 to C3b by substances such as endotoxin. Increased capillary permeability is largely due to the release of histamine from mast cells in response to C3a and C5a. These factors are also chemotactic for neutrophils. Lysis of cells coated with complement is a function of the late complement components C8 and C9, which create holes in cell membranes. Heat treatment is the standard laboratory method for inactivating complement.

4. IgM rheumatoid factor

- ☐ A indicates disease when present
- ☐ B is not useful for monitoring treatment
- ☐ C reacts with the Fc component of IgG
- ☐ D is positive in infective endocarditis
- ☐ E is positive in 50% of patients with rheumatoid nodules

5. In systemic lupus erythematosus

- ☐ A the C reactive protein (CRP) is raised
- ☐ B the lymphocyte count is raised
- ☐ C the platelet count can be low
- ☐ D marrow hypoplasia is seen
- ☐ E there is no increase risk of thrombosis

6. Among the features of systemic lupus erythematosus

- ☐ A joint disease is characteristically non-erosive
- ☐ B Raynaud's disease is uncommon
- ☐ C livedo reticularis is pathognomonic
- ☐ D subacute cutaneous disease is usually benign
- ☐ E hypertension is common

Answers overleaf

4. B C D

Around 70% of all rheumatoid arthritis patients, and 100% of those with nodules, are sero-positive for IgM rheumatoid factor. Secreted by B cells, the IgM factor reacts with the Fc component of IgG. The Rose-Waaler test uses sheep red cells coated with rabbit IgG. IgM factor is not specific to rheumatoid arthritis and may be seen in other disease and chronic infection.

5. C D

Autoantibodies can cause a haemolytic anaemia, neutropenia, lymphopenia, or thrombocytopenia; the bone marrow is usually hypercellular but may be aplastic as a consequence of treatment. The CRP is usually normal and if raised may suggest sepsis. Other investigations show raised levels of immunoglobulins and a reduced complement. Antiphospholipid/anticardiolipin antibodies are found in some cases of SLE and are prothrombotic.

6. A D E

Joint disease is characteristically non-erosive. Raynaud's disease is a feature in 50% of cases. Livido reticularis can be found in several conditions including bronchial and pancreatic carcinoma and polyarteritis nodosa. Hypertension and renal disease should be treated vigorously.

7. The following statements are true:

- ☐ A occipital headaches can occur in temporal arteritis
- ☐ B corneal reflex loss may be an early sign of rheumatoid cervical myelopathy
- ☐ C the nail-fold infarcts of rheumatoid vasculitis represent evidence of a life-threatening complication
- ☐ D iron therapy is effective in correcting the anaemia of rheumatoid arthritis
- ☐ E gold injections are usually given intra-articularly

8. The antiphospholipid syndrome

- ☐ A is associated with arterial thrombosis
- ☐ B may cause a chorea
- ☐ C is treated with high dose warfarin
- ☐ D only occurs in association with SLE
- ☐ E can cause sudden wide spread organ failure

9. Carpal tunnel syndrome

- ☐ A may present with pain in the forearm
- ☐ B is associated with fasciculation of the small muscles of the hand
- ☐ C is exacerbated by coughing and sneezing
- ☐ D an underlying medical condition is usually present
- ☐ E is common in diffuse eosinophilic fascitis

Answers overleaf

7. A B

The occipital artery may be involved as well as the temporal in temporal arteritis. The loss of the corneal reflex is due to compression of the spinal tract of the Vth cranial nerve which reaches to the level of the atlanto-axial joint of the neck. Nail-fold vasculitis is benign and self-limiting. Iron therapy is ineffective, and may make inflammation worse. Gold is given intramuscularly.

8. A B C E

Antiphospholipid and anticardiolipin antibodies are found in 5% of the general population and in association with several connective tissue vasculitides, infection and malignancy. Arterial and venous thrombosis and spontaneous abortion are classic features but skin disorders and CNS abnormalities are increasingly described. A 'catastrophic' variant leads to multiple organ failure with widespread thrombosis. The treatment of recurrent disease is high dose warfarin at an INR of 3–4.

9. A E

The pain of median nerve compression can radiate to the forearm and may even present as a painful shoulder. Fasciculation is not a feature especially not of the small muscles of the hand as they are innervated by the ulnar nerve. Exacerbation by raising CSF pressure on coughing suggests nerve root compression in the neck. An underlying condition is rarely present in practice: most cases occurring in middle-aged people are a combination of hardening of the flexor retinaculum plus a congenitally small tunnel.

10. In the vasculitides

- ☐ A cANCA has a high sensitivity for Wegener's granulomatosis
- ☐ B neurological symptoms are a common feature of Churg–Straus
- ☐ C the pathological hall mark of Henoch-Schönlein purpura (HSP) is IgG in the skin and renal messangium
- ☐ D microscopic polyangiitis is more common in women
- ☐ E glomerulonephritis is a common feature of polyarteritis nodosa

11. Secondary (reactive) amyloidosis

- ☐ A results from an inability to mount an acute phase response
- ☐ B causes ulceration of the tongue
- ☐ C characteristically presents as a glomerulonephritis
- ☐ D only complicates rheumatic diseases in adults
- ☐ E can be reversed by controlling the underlying disease

12. The following statements about the spondylo-arthropathies are correct:

- ☐ A tissue typing for HLA-B27 is particularly useful
- ☐ B they are more common in adult males
- ☐ C transient disease is often non-erosive
- ☐ D anterior uveitis occurs in 30% of patients
- ☐ E sacro-iliitis can be unilateral or bilateral

Answers overleaf

10. A

A positive cANCA is sensitive for Wegener's granulomatosis. Both Wegener's granulomatosis and microscopic polyangiitis are more common in men and associated with pulmonary–renal disease. ENT symptoms are an important feature of Wegener's granulomatosis. Churg–Strauss patients rarely have neurological complications. Biopsy in HSP shows IgA deposits. Polyarteritis nodosa is associated with renal disease due to thrombosis, infarction or aneurysms and necrotising arteritis.

11. None are correct

Reactive amyloidosis occurs as a result of a prolonged acute phase response, particularly elevation of the serum amyloid A protein which in genetically predisposed individuals cannot be catabolised and so becomes deposited in tissues as fibrils. The tongue may be enlarged with amyloid but not ulcerated. It typically presents with nephrotic syndrome. It may occur in children as well as adults and is progressive and fatal despite good control of the underlying disease.

12. B C E

HLA-B27 is not usually helpful or reliable prognostically. The spondyloarthropathies can occur at any age but do so most often in young adults; spinal symptoms are more common in men. Synovitis is indistinguishable from that of rheumatoid arthritis but has a better prognosis and if transient is non-erosive. Eye lesions include conjunctivitis in 30% of patients with a 'reactive' arthritis but the overall incidence of uveitis generally is 5%. The iliitis of ankylosing spondylitis tends to be bilateral and that of psoriasis and Reiter's disease can be unilateral.

13. Interleukin-1 (IL-1)

☐ A is a lymphocyte activating factor
☐ B is an endogenous pyrogen
☐ C inhibits fibroblast proliferation
☐ D stimulates the synthesis of acute phase proteins in the liver
☐ E is not synthesised by macrophages

14. Raynauds phenomenon

☐ A is much more common in women
☐ B is a feature of Sjögren's syndrome
☐ C can be treated with ACE-inhibitors
☐ D is due to blood vessel hyper-reactivity
☐ E affects 5–10% of the population

15. The following statements about synovial fluid are true:

☐ A it is often blood-stained in acute pyrophosphate arthropathy
☐ B the greater the inflammation, the more viscous the fluid
☐ C a turbid fluid indicates the presence of infection
☐ D synovial fluid lactate levels are higher in infected than in non-infected effusions
☐ E crystals may be visualised by holding a specimen against a dark background in natural daylight

Answers overleaf

13. A B C D

IL-1 has many biological effects including A, B, and D. IL-1 also is chemotactic for lymphocytes, increases the thrombogenicity of the endothelial luminal surface, promotes leucocyte adhesion to endothelium by an action on endothelial cells, and stimulates fibroblast proliferation. IL-1 is synthesised by many cells, of which macrophages are amongst the most important. Other sources include Langerhans cells, dendritic cells, keratinocytes and endothelial cells.

14. A B C D E

There is a strong (90%) female predominance. It is relatively rare in rheumatoid arthritis, but is common in SLE and Sjögren's disease. In scleroderma, Raynaud's phenomenon and nail fold capillary abnormalities with a positive ANA is a finding in 90% of cases destined to develop full systemic sclerosis. Treatment options include calcium channel blockers, ACE-inhibitors, gamolenic acid, prostacyclin and sympathectomy.

15. A D

Synovial inflammation is associated with release of proteolytic enzymes which degrade the hyaluronate making the fluid less viscous. A turbid fluid indicates the presence of white cells, not necessarily infection. Raised lactate levels are found in septic arthritis. Crystals of pyrophosphate and urate can be seen using polarised light microscopy. They are not visible to the naked eye.

16. The delayed hypersensitivity reaction (Type IV)

- ☐ A is a humoral immune response
- ☐ B is dependent upon T lymphocytes
- ☐ C is characterised by a mononuclear cell infiltration
- ☐ D is caused by deposition of immune complexes in tissues
- ☐ E is mediated by IgE antibodies bound to Fc receptors on mast cells and basophil granulocytes

17. Features of Behçet's disease include

- ☐ A central nervous system disorders
- ☐ B erythema nodosum
- ☐ C venous thrombosis in 75% of patients
- ☐ D iritis
- ☐ E diarrhoea

18. In septic arthritis

- ☐ A a Gram stain should be done immediately
- ☐ B turbidity of the aspirate implies infection
- ☐ C clinical suspicion of Lyme disease would lead a clinician to chose tetracycline for 'blind' therapy
- ☐ D rubella is accompanied by a self-limiting polyarthropathy
- ☐ E beta haemolytic *Strep.* accounts for 50% of all cases

Answers overleaf

16. B C

The delayed type hypersensitivity reaction (Type IV) is a T cell mediated response that results in a mononuclear cell infiltration into the site of antigen deposition. The cutaneous response to tuberculin purified protein derivative (PPD) is a typical example. Humoral antibodies are involved in types II and III hypersensitivity. In type II hypersensitivity, autoantibodies are directed against cell surface antigens, as in autoimmune haemolytic anaemia. In type III hypersensitivity, immune complexes are deposited in tissues, either in antibody excess (e.g. Farmer's lung) or in antigen excess (e.g. serum sickness). E refers to immediate (type I) hypersensitivity.

17. A B D E

Behçet's disease is twice as common in males. The mean age of onset is 30 years. The other important clinical feature is oro-genital ulceration. Venous thrombosis occurs in around 25% of cases. It is associated with HLA B5. Steroids and cyclosporin A are used in treatment.

18. A D

Aspiration of a suspected septic joint should be followed immediately by antibiotics pending a Gram stain and culture. A high white cell count and turbidity is non-specific; a high lactate suggests infection. *Staphylococcus aureus* accounts for 50% of infection; beta haemolytic *Streptococcus* 10%. The skin lesions of Lyme disease are best treated with tetracycline but the septic arthritis requires intravenous penicillin. About 20% of women with rubella can have a self-limiting, 'rheumatoid' like polyarthropathy which subsides after 6–8 weeks.

19. Sjögren's syndrome

☐ A should be treated with topical steroid eye drops

☐ B causes dyspareunia

☐ C affects men more than women

☐ D may cause facial swelling

☐ E is associated with the Anti-SS-A antibody

20. In the crystal arthropathies

☐ A acute gout is treated with uricosuric drugs

☐ B blood urate is a reliable test for confirming gout

☐ C all patients with hyperuricaemia should receive allopurinol

☐ D hyperparathyroidism is associated with pseudo-gout

☐ E the absence of chondrocalcinosis on X-ray rules out a diagnosis of pseudo-gout

21. Osteomalacia

☐ A is associated with a myopathy

☐ B causes reduced bone volume

☐ C must be corrected by using the more potent forms of vitamin D such as 1-alpha hydroxycholecalciferol

☐ D may result in tertiary hyperparathyroidism

☐ E causes lesions that are undetectable on bone scintigraphy

Answers overleaf

19. B D E

Steroid eye drops are not required and may be dangerous by predisposing to infection (particularly as a dry eye is prone to bacterial and fungal infection), scleral softening and perforation. The eye should be kept moist by regular use of artificial tears. Patients with some tear flow may benefit from electrocoagulation of the nasolacrimal glands to encourage the accumulation of residual tear drops. Other exocrine secretions, including those of the vagina, are affected, and the salivary glands may be enlarged typically in unilateral and episodic fashion. Most patients have the Anti-SS-A antibody named after the 'A' antigen of Sjögren's syndrome, now called anti-Ro.

20. D

Acute gout is treated with NSAIDs or colchicine. Aspirin, allopurinol and probenecid should be avoided initially. Blood urate corresponds poorly with clinical symptoms of gout and can be normal during an attack and raised in the asymptomatic; in this respect, hyperuricaemia *per se* is not an indication for allopurinol. Increased urate production is found in myeloproliferative disorders, high purine intake, obesity and excess alcohol and fructose consumption. A reduction in excretion is seen in intrinsic renal disease, with excess of metabolites (ketones, lactate) and with the use of thiazide diuretics. The causes of chondrocalcinosis include hypothyroidism, hypomagnesaemia, hypophosphatasia and haemochromatosis.

21. A D

Muscle weakness and tenderness are quite common and may contribute to the characteristic waddling gait. The bone volume is normal but undercalcified. The more potent forms of vitamin D are not required since uncomplicated osteomalacia is due to dietary deficiency and is therefore not resistant to treatment. The potent forms can be dangerous resulting in hypercalcaemia. Prolonged hypocalcaemia results in secondary hyperparathyroidism which can occasionally become autonomous. The bone scan is a useful way of detecting lesions since the decalcified bones avidly take up bone-seeking isotopes.

22. Leucocytes of the CD4 T4 phenotype

- ☐ A are lymphocytes
- ☐ B do not recirculate
- ☐ C are phagocytic
- ☐ D are infected by the Human Immunodeficiency Virus (HIV)
- ☐ E perform a 'helper' role in the on-going immune response

23. In Paget's disease

- ☐ A the alkaline phosphatase is always raised and a good marker of bone turnover
- ☐ B the characteristic early lesion is a resorption front of abnormally large osteoclasts
- ☐ C all bisphosphonates directly inhibit osteoblastic activity at therapeutic dose
- ☐ D spread to other bones is a late feature of the disease
- ☐ E paraparesis may occur

24. Anti-histone antibodies

- ☐ A are associated with thrombosis
- ☐ B are found in the absence of antibodies to native DNA in drug induced SLE
- ☐ C are associated with congenital heart block
- ☐ D are a marker for polymyositis
- ☐ E are not found in rheumatoid arthritis

Answers overleaf

22. A D E

The T4 antigen, now designated CD4 (CD=cluster of differentiation), is a marker for a subpopulation of T lymphocytes that are thought to play a 'helper' role in the immune response. Long-lived resting lymphocytes enter lymphoid tissue, such as lymph nodes, pass through the lymphoid parenchyma into efferent lymph. Thence the lymphocytes pass into the central lymphatic ducts and then back into the blood stream. This process of lymphocyte migration is called recirculation and allows each individual lymphoid organ to share the large pool of recirculating lymphocytes with the rest of the immune system, thus disseminating immunological function and memory. Most small resting T lymphocytes are considered to be recirculating cells. HIV preferentially infects T4 cells and may enter the cell by way of the T4 antigen.

23. B E

The initial pathology in Paget's disease is abnormal resorption. Osteoclasts, via cytokines, stimulate osteoblastic remineralisation but the new bone architecture is not normal. Alkaline phosphatase (ALP) and hydroxyproline are good markers of bone turnover but ALP is not always raised in symptomatic patients. It is very rare to find new bone involvement after the initial diagnosis other than some spread along those bones already affected.The bisphosphonates are analogues of pyrophosphate and inhibit osteoclastic activity. Etidronate in high doses can inhibit osteoblasts and induce osteomalacia.

24. B

Although anti-histone antibodies are found in 30-80% of sera from patients with idiopathic SLE, their presence in patients with clinical SLE who lack antibodies to native DNA is suggestive of a drug induced syndrome. Anti-histone antibodies are found in 15-20% of patients with rheumatoid arthritis and are therefore only diagnostically valuable in the appropriate clinical setting. A refers to anti-cardiolipin antibodies. C refers to antibodies to the Ro (SS-A) antigen. D refers to antibodies to the Jo-1 antigen.

25. The following statements about endocrinopathies are correct:

- ☐ A hypoparathyroidism is associated with osteoporosis
- ☐ B hyperparathyroidism produces features of ligament calcification similar to ankylosing spondylitis
- ☐ C acute pseudogout is a feature of acromegaly
- ☐ D diabetes mellitus is associated with 'hypertrophic ankylosing hyperostosis' (Forestiers disease)
- ☐ E the soft tissue swelling of thyroid acropachy responds to treatment of the underlying thyrotoxicosis

26. The following statements are true:

- ☐ A radiological sacroiliitis is characteristically unilateral in ankylosing spondylitis
- ☐ B periostitis is a frequent radiological finding in psoriatic arthropathy
- ☐ C juxta-articular osteoporosis does not occur with gouty erosions
- ☐ D erosions are characteristically periarticular in systemic lupus erythematosus (SLE)
- ☐ E gouty tophi are radio-opaque

27. Reiters syndrome

- ☐ A is the most common cause of an inflammatory oligoarthropathy in young men
- ☐ B is characterised by uveitis
- ☐ C is associated with buccal ulceration
- ☐ D is most often self limiting
- ☐ E disease activity correlates well with the ESR

Answers overleaf

25. C D

Hyperparathyroidism is associated with gout, pseudo-gout and osteoporosis; hypoparathyroidism can produce a picture similar to ankylosing spondylitis. Forestiers disease and cheiroarthropathy (pseudo-scleroderma) are features of diabetes mellitis.

26. B C

Sacroiliitis is characteristically bilateral and symmetrical in ankylosing spondylitis. Unilateral, asymmetrical involvement is more common in other forms of seronegative spondarthritis such as psoriasis and Reiter's syndrome. Fluffy periostitis often occurs in conjunction with erosions in psoriatic arthropathy, so-called proliferative erosions. SLE is a non-erosive arthropathy and although there may be considerable hand deformity, this is due to tendon involvement rather than joint destruction. Gouty tophi do not calcify as a rule and are therefore radiolucent. The bone density around gouty erosions is usually normal although during an acute attack of gout there may be osteoporosis in the affected joint.

27. C

The triad of urethritis, conjunctivitis and arthritis is characteristic; added to this is buccal ulceration and balanitis and 20% have sacro-iliitis. About 1% of patients with a non-specific urethritis develop Reiter's syndrome. The disease is often not self-limiting and may progress with 80% of patients having symptoms at 5 years.

28. The following are characteristically involved:

- ☐ A the MCP joints in psoriatic arthropathy
- ☐ B the hip in ankylosing spondylitis
- ☐ C the DIP joints in pyrophosphate arthropathy
- ☐ D the MTP joints in haemophilia
- ☐ E the hand and foot in sickle cell disease

29. The causes of osteomalacia include

- ☐ A primary biliary cirrhosis
- ☐ B Fanconi syndrome
- ☐ C acute renal failure
- ☐ D renal tubular acidosis
- ☐ E primary hyperparathyroidism

30. The following statements on osteogenesis imperfecta are correct:

- ☐ A blue sclera are common to all types
- ☐ B the condition is autosomal recessive
- ☐ C hearing loss is mainly conductive
- ☐ D aortic incompetence is a feature
- ☐ E the biochemical disorder is of type II collagen

Answers overleaf

28. B E

There are several characteristic patterns of joint involvement in psoriasis: 1. DIP joint disease in association with nail dystrophy (10%); 2. asymmetrical oligoarticular involvement of the small distal joints (70%); 3. symmetrical polyarthritis (15%); 4. axial with spondylitis as a major feature (5%); 5. arthritis mutilans (rare). Generally, a seronegative oligoarthritis with DIP and PIP involvement with relative sparing of the MCP joints suggests a diagnosis of psoriatic arthritis. Extraspinal joint involvement occurs in 40% of patients with ankylosing spondylitis, the hip and knee being the commonest sites. Pyrophosphate deposition occurs mainly in the large joints, particularly the knees, wrists and shoulders. The joints involved in haemophilia (in order of frequency) are the knee, elbow, ankle, shoulder, wrist and sternoclavicular joint. Acute pain and swelling of a digit or a whole extremity is characteristic of multiple bone infarction in children during a sickle crisis.

29. A B D E

Privational causes include food fads and poor diet intake of vitamin D. Gastrointestinal disturbances including gastrectomy, malabsorption and liver disease can all lead to osteomalacia. The renal tubular diseases have high phosphate clearance in common and chronic renal failure (not acute) leads to a decreased production of 1,25 dihydroxy vitamin D.

30. C D

Osteogenesis imperfecta (OI) occurs in 1 in 30,000 births. It is a disorder of bone type I collagen and all except type III OI are autosomal dominant. Type I and IV OI are the more common variants and relatively benign; type IV have normal sclerae. Type III OI is associated with progressive severe disease and multiple fractures. Type II is non-viable. Other features include abnormal dentine and ossicles, hypermobility, tendon rupture and leaky heart valves.

31. The following are secondary causes of osteoporosis:

- ☐ A Klinefelter's syndrome
- ☐ B Cushing's disease
- ☐ C frusemide
- ☐ D multiple myeloma
- ☐ E acromegaly

32. The following are characteristic of polymyalgia rheumatica (PMR):

- ☐ A depression
- ☐ B weight loss
- ☐ C lymphadenopathy
- ☐ D raised muscle enzymes
- ☐ E sternoclavicular joint swelling

33. In disorders of phosphate metabolism

- ☐ A the most common cause of hypophosphataemia is chronic renal failure
- ☐ B hyperphosphataemia complicates hypoparathyroidism
- ☐ C hypophosphataemia is a feature of Fanconi syndrome
- ☐ D hypoxia is associated with severe hypophosphataemia
- ☐ E tetany is a feature of hyperphosphataemia

Answers overleaf

31. A B C D E

Several endocrinopathies can cause osteoporosis; others to consider are thyrotoxicosis, hyperparathyroidism and hypogonadism. Other drugs associated with the condition are steroids, heparin and cytotoxics. Conditions such as myeloma lead to osteoporosis partly by a local infiltrative affect but also by cytokine stimulation of bone resorption.

32. A B E

The typical features of PMR outside the musculoskeletal system are depression and weight loss. There may also be low-grade fever. If temporal arteritis supervenes there may also be headache and facial pain. The presence of lymphadenopathy should alert one to the possibility of a paraneoplastic syndrome, which may present with similar clinical features. Muscle enzymes are raised in polymyositis which is associated with muscle fibril destruction. It is increasingly recognised that there may be synovitis in patients with PMR particularly affecting the shoulders and sternoclavicular joints. Occasionally there may also be peripheral synovitis in the small joints of the hands resembling rheumatoid arthritis.

33. B C D E

Dietary phosphate is absorbed (both active and passive) throughout the small bowel, mostly from the jejunum. The kidney responds immediately to changes in serum phosphate levels and normally over 90% of the filtered load is reabsorbed from the proximal tubules. Chronic renal failure is the most common cause of hyperphosphataemia; raised levels are also found in hypoparathyroidism, hyperthyroidism, acromegaly, tumoral calcinosis and with bisphosphonate therapy. An increased phosphate load may be a feature of vitamin D toxicity, cytotoxic therapy and rhabdomyolysis. Renal phosphate wasting is seen in Fanconi's syndrome and ketoacidosis; other causes of hypophosphataemia include alcoholism and the administration of glucose and insulin. High levels of phosphate lead to hypocalcaemia and tetany; very low levels result in 2,3 DPG and tissue ATP deficiency and associated haemolytic anaemia and muscle weakness.

IMMUNOLOGY

Mark your answers with a tick (True) or a cross (False) in the box provided. Leave the box blank for 'Don't know'.

34. The following statements on cellular immunity are correct:

☐ A cytotoxic T cells (CTL) carry CD8 glycoprotein and respond to peptides presented by HLA class 1

☐ B CTL produce interleukin 2 (IL-2)

☐ C Di George syndrome is associated with impaired cellular immunity

☐ D lymphopenia is a feature of ataxia telangiectasia

☐ E Wiscott–Aldrich disease is an autosomal recessive condition characterised by depressed cellular immunity

35. Of the complement pathway

☐ A the liver is a site of complement component synthesis

☐ B factor B is cleaved by factor H forming a stable C3bBb complex in the 'alternative' pathway

☐ C the 'alternative' pathway positive-feedback loop is controlled by factor I

☐ D single IgG antibody-immune complex is the most efficient stimulant of the 'classical' pathway

☐ E C2 component deficiency is the most common isolated deficiency of complement among Caucasians

36. In cytokine production and function

☐ A tumour necrosis factor (TNF) alpha is mainly produced by T lymphocytes

☐ B interferon (IFN) gamma has a strong antiviral action by inducing biochemical adaptation in infected cells

☐ C interleukin 1 (IL-1) induces prostaglandin synthesis

☐ D transforming growth factor (TGF) beta inhibits the acute inflammatory response

☐ E interleukin 2 (IL-2) stimulates the growth and differentiation of B cells

Answers overleaf

34. A C D

T helper cells (Th) express CD4 and recognise HLA (major histocompatibility complex) class 2. Most CTL are CD8+ and restricted to class 1 HLA. A sub-class of Th cells produce IL-2. Di George syndrome (thymic aplasia) is associated with impaired T cell production. Immunoglobulin levels are usually adequate and there is an increased risk of autoimmune disease. Ataxia telangiectasia has several deficiencies of immunoglobulins and lymphopenia; it is autosomal recessive. Wiscott–Aldrich syndrome is X-linked, the gene defect leading to abnormalities in the regulation of sialophorin (CD43). The condition is characterised by thrombocytopenia and lymphopenia.

35. A C E

Via the alternative pathway, Bb (cleaved from factor B by factor D) binds to C3b to form the unstable C3bBb (equivalent to C3 convertase of the classical pathway). The compound is then stabalised by properidin. C3-nephritic factor (found in some cases of membrano-proliferative GN type II) is an autoantibody that stabilises C3bBb; the positive feedback amplification of the alternative pathway cascade then consumes C3 (but not C4). Factor H can bind to C3b and, by acting as a cofactor, allows factor I to inactive C3b, controlling further activation of the pathway. The classical pathway is activated by antigen–antibody complexes binding to multiple domain C1q; the pentameric head of IgM makes this the most efficient stimulant.

36. C D E

The cytokine family includes interleukins, TNF, IFN, colony stimulating factors, growth factors and chemokines. TNF-alpha is mainly produced by macrophages. It regulates cell growth and stimulates leucocytes and the induction of adhesion receptors. TNF-beta is produced by T cells. IFN-alpha and IFN-beta induce biochemical adaptation in uninfected cells, increasing protection against viral invasion. IFN-gamma has little antiviral action in this way and is more important in regulating cell-mediated immunity. IL-1 and IL-2 stimulate both B and T cells; IL-1 also stimulates prostaglandin synthesis. TGF-beta promotes humoral rather than cellular immunity and appears to reduce the intensity of the acute inflammatory reaction.

37. The following are diseases with specific defects in phagocyte function:

- ☐ A myeloperoxidase deficiency
- ☐ B purine nucleoside phosphorylase deficiency
- ☐ C Job's syndrome
- ☐ D Chediak–Higashi syndrome
- ☐ E Bloom's syndrome

38. The following statements are correct:

- ☐ A IgA can activate complement via the alternative pathway
- ☐ B IgA normally represents less than 1% of the serum immunoglobulin pool
- ☐ C J-chains are associated with both IgA and IgM
- ☐ D the Fab fragment determines the class of immunoglobulin
- ☐ E IgE can cross the placenta

39. The following HLA associations are correct:

- ☐ A HLA DR3 and dermatitis herpetiformis
- ☐ B HLA A3 and schizophrenia
- ☐ C HLA DR2 and Goodpasture's syndrome
- ☐ D HLA DQW2 and coeliac disease
- ☐ E HLA DR7 and Hashimoto's thyroiditis

40. In the metabolism of arachidonic acid

- ☐ A arachidonic acid is converted to leukotrienes via phospholipase A2
- ☐ B corticosteroids inhibit phospholipase A2
- ☐ C 5-lipoxygenase is blocked by aspirin
- ☐ D platelets are a major source of leukotrienes
- ☐ E non-steroidal anti-inflammatory drugs with a high cyclo-oxygenase type 1 (COX 1) to type 2 (COX2) activity ratio may have fewer gastrointestinal side-effects

Answers overleaf

37. A C D

Conditions B and E are associated with T cell abnormalities. Neutrophil chemotaxis and lysosome formation are defective in Job's syndrome and Chediak–Higashi syndrome respectively.

38. A C

Secretory IgA is dimeric, the two subunits joined by a J-chain; IgM is pentameric. IgA and IgE can fix complement via the alternative pathway; IgG and IgM via the classical pathway. Of the normal total immunoglobulin pool IgG makes up approx 75%, IgA 15% and IgM 10%. There are traces of IgD and IgE. Only IgG can cross the placenta. The constant region of the molecule (Fc) determines the class of immunoglobulin. The Fab region has a variable (V) and constant (CH) domain, the former being unique for each antibody.

39. A C D

Certain HLA alleles are associated with increased risk of disease. The following are further examples: A3/B14 in haemochromatosis; A28 in schizophrenia; B5 in Behçet's disease and ulcerative colitis; DR3/7 DQW2 in coeliac disease; B27 in ankylosing spondylitis and psoriatic arthropathy; DR2 in Goodpasture's syndrome and narcolepsy; DR3 in chronic active hepatitis, Grave's disease, myasthenia gravis, Addison's disease and Sjögren's syndrome; DR4 in rheumatoid arthritis and insulin dependent diabetes, and DR5 in Hashimoto's thyroiditis.

40. B

Esterified fatty acids are converted to arachidonic acid via phospholipase A2; this reaction is inhibited by corticosteroids. Arachidonic acid is then converted to leukotrienes via 5-lipoxygenase, and prostaglandins via cyclo-oxygenase. NSAIDs block prostaglandin synthesis. Two subtypes of COX have been identified. COX 1 activation leads to the production of prostacyclin, is antithrombogenic and cytoprotective in the gastric mucosa. It is now thought that the inhibition of inflammation by NSAIDs is mostly a consequence of inhibiting COX2 and that the inhibition of COX1 leads to gastric side-effects; thus NSAID with high COX2 to COX1 activity ratio (selective COX2 inhibition) may have good anti-inflammatory action with fewer side-effects.

HAEMATOLOGY

Mark your answers with a tick (True) or a cross (False) in the box provided. Leave the box blank for 'Don't know'.

41. In idiopathic thrombocytopenic purpura (ITP)

- ☐ A most cases are due to an immune mediated destruction of platelets
- ☐ B if the spleen is palpable then the thrombocytopenia is likely to be due to another cause
- ☐ C maternal anti-platelet antibodies may cause neonatal thrombocytopenia
- ☐ D the disease usually becomes chronic when it presents in childhood
- ☐ E the disease is associated with HIV infection

42. In chronic granulocytic leukaemia (CGL)

- ☐ A a 9:22 chromosome translocation is necessary to establish the diagnosis
- ☐ B transformation into myelofibrosis may occur
- ☐ C development of further chromosome abnormalities heralds a change in the character of the disease
- ☐ D busulphan therapy delays the onset of blast transformation
- ☐ E bone marrow transplantation in the chronic phase may be curative

43. After splenectomy

- ☐ A Howell–Jolly bodies are found in the red cells
- ☐ B there is an exaggerated neutrophil and platelet response to inflammation
- ☐ C penicillin prophylaxis against staphylococcal infection should be continued for life
- ☐ D lymphopenia is found
- ☐ E meningococcal vaccine should be administered to patients visiting equatorial Africa

Answers overleaf

41. A B C E

Although termed ‘idiopathic’ most cases are due to coating of the platelets with anti-platelet antibodies. Platelet surface immunoglobulin tests may be positive but these tests are technically demanding and there may be too few platelets to do them. Although the spleen may be enlarged on scan, it is rarely palpable. Children usually have an acute self-limiting form of the disease. A history of i.v. drug abuse or HIV exposure should be sought in all males presenting with ITP.

42. B C E

Approximately 5% of cases lack the characteristic Philadelphia chromosome: many of these cases do have the associated bor:abl hybrid gene if investigated by PCR. Most cases transform into a blast crisis though a few do become myelofibiotic. Patients under the age of 45 should receive transplants if they have an HLA matched suitable sibling donor. If aged under 25 then a matched unrelated donor should be sought from the national panels such as the Anthony Nolan.

43. A B E

Howell–Jolly bodies are nuclear remnants usually removed from red cells (pitted) by the spleen; they are the most obvious feature of a post-splenectomy blood film. Target cells, occasional spherocytes and red cell anisocytosis are found and some patients have a lymphocytosis. Current recommendations are that all patients having splenectomy should have pneumococcal and Hib vaccines before splenectomy and life-long penicillin prophylaxis against pneumococcus and meningococcus. When visiting malarial areas they should have meticulous chemoprophylaxis.

44. The following are features of myelodysplastic syndrome:

- ☐ A increased numbers of blasts in the bone marrow
- ☐ B atypical monocytes in the peripheral blood
- ☐ C transfusion-dependent anaemia
- ☐ D transformation into treatment-resistant acute myeloid leukaemia (AML)
- ☐ E treatment with busulphan may be effective

45. In acute leukaemia

- ☐ A the presence of Auer rods confirms the diagnosis of acute lymphoblastic leukaemia (ALL)
- ☐ B the presence of the Philadelphia chromosome confers a good prognosis
- ☐ C disseminated intravascular coagulation (DIC) is common in acute promyelocytic leukaemia (AML-M3)
- ☐ D CNS involvement is common in acute lymphoblastic leukaemia
- ☐ E hypokalaemia in acute monocytic leukaemia is due to renal tubular damage by lysozyme

46. When giving a blood transfusion

- ☐ A administration of Rhesus positive blood to a Rhesus positive recipient can be followed by haemolytic problems due to Rhesus-group antibiodies
- ☐ B a fever in the recipient developing during transfusion is an indication to stop transfusing
- ☐ C using stored blood, the oxygen delivering capacity of the blood is not restored until about 2 days later
- ☐ D with stored blood, one can assume that no viable white blood cells remain 24 hours after the blood donation
- ☐ E CMV antibody-negative blood should be used for all recipients who are themselves CMV negative

Answers overleaf

44. A B C D

This heterogeneous group of conditions is usually characterised by transfusion-dependent, or 'refractory' anaemia. The presence of 5–20% of blasts in the marrow is seen in refractory anaemia with excess of blasts. A proportion of patients transform into resistant AML, with a marrow blast count >30%. A more indolent condition associated with atypical monocytes in the peripheral blood and marrow has been labelled 'chronic myelomonocytic leukaemia'. Treatment of these conditions with cytotoxic drugs prior to the development of frank leukaemia is of doubtful value. Busulphan is of value in the myeloproliferative disorders, not in this group of conditions.

45. C D E

Auer rods are a diagnostic feature of acute myeloid leukaemia. Philadelphia chromosome carries a poor prognosis whether found in AML or ALL. Release of procoagulant granules before and during treatment of acute promyelocytic leukaemia may cause acute DIC, frequently associated with increased fibrinolysis. Many units give prophylactic tranexamic acid. Monocytic leukaemia is also associated with gum hypertrophy.

46. A

The term Rhesus positive refers to patients whose red cells bear the antigen D and does not take account of the other antigens in the Rhesus group. Thus Rhesus positive blood which is commonly CDe/cde may induce antibody formation against C, c or e if the recipient does not possess these antigens. Fever may develop during transfusion due to non-specific pyrogens or to WBC or platelet antibodies in patients who have received previous transfusions; it is safe to continue as long as no additional signs and symptoms develop. 2,3 diphosphoglycerate is reduced in stored red cells, but is restored 4–12 hours after transfusion thus restoring oxygen delivering capacity. Dextran can cause RBC agglutination *in vitro* and so complicate the cross-match reaction. It does not cause clinical problems. Lymphocytes remain viable in stored blood for several days and can cause graft versus host disease in severely immuno-compromised recipients. CMV-negative blood is only required for CMV-negative recipients who are immuno-compromised for example marrow transplantation.

47. Fragmented red cells on the blood film

- ☐ A are found in disseminated intravascular coagulation
- ☐ B in thrombotic thrombocytopenic purpura are due to damage to red cells by intravascular fibrin
- ☐ C are found in march haemoglobinuria
- ☐ D are usually associated with polychromasia
- ☐ E are associated with increased serum haptoglobins.

48. The following are features of iron-deficiency anaemia:

- ☐ A reduced bone marrow stainable iron
- ☐ B reduced serum iron and iron binding capacity (TIBC)
- ☐ C a low MCV, MCH and MCHC
- ☐ D target cells and pencil cells in the peripheral blood
- ☐ E correction can almost always be achieved with simple oral iron preparations

49. Vitamin B12

- ☐ A deficiency causes malabsorption
- ☐ B intramuscular administration of more than 1 mg/week results in haemolysis
- ☐ C serum levels are increased in polycythaemia rubra vera
- ☐ D the presence of intrinsic factor antibodies provides strong supportive evidence for the diagnosis of pernicious anaemia
- ☐ E hydroxocobalamin is derived from liver extract

Answers overleaf

47. A B D

The features of a microangiopathic haemolytic blood picture are fragmented cells and helmet cells with polychromasia and increased reticulocyte count. The red cells are damaged by contact with fibrin in the small blood vessels. The fibrin strands may be laid down in disseminated intravascular coagulation or any cause of inflammation of the small blood vessels such as vasculitis, or glomerulonephritis. Rare causes are thrombotic thrombocytopenic purpura and haemolytic uraemic syndrome. Free haemoglobin released into the plasma is bound to haptoglobin in order to prevent loss of haemoglobin in the urine. Levels of haptoglobin will be reduced in intravascular haemolysis. When haptoglobins are used up haemoglobin will bind to albumin, forming methaemalbumin which may be detected in the blood by the Schumm's test, a useful test for intravascular haemolysis. Release of more haemoglobin results in haemoglobinuria.

48. C D E

Iron stores in the marrow have to be non-existent before any alteration in the haemoglobin occurs; thereafter anaemia follows. Serum iron is reduced, but the TIBC increases, so that the TIBC is less than 10% saturated Fe/TIBC >1/10. The red cells are small, with reduced cell content and concentration, giving rise to the 'microcytic hypochromic' film which together with anisocytosis, target cells and pencil cells makes the classical iron deficiency picture. Oral iron is nearly always adequate; if the anaemia fails to respond, one should consider continued blood loss, severe malabsorption, poor compliance or a wrong initial diagnosis. Ferrous sulphate is the cheapest and most effective preparation, 'slow release' formulations release iron into the lower small bowel from which it is poorly absorbed.

49. A C D

All rapidly dividing cells require B12 and folic acid, including the lining of the intestinal tract, so patients with deficiency often complain of sore mouths and mild diarrhoea and have a malabsorption type Schilling test result if this investigation is done too early in the treatment of the disease. Vitamin B12 is cheap and non-toxic, it may be given daily during the first week of treatment. In the myeloproliferative disorders the increased numbers of developing myeloid cells produce increased amounts of B12 binding protein, increasing the serum level. This may be a useful marker for myeloproliferative disorders. Parietal cell antibodies have a low diagnostic specificity for pernicious anaemia, being found in half of women over 60, but intrinsic factor antibodies are more useful. Hydroxocobalamin is derived from bacterial fermentation and may be given to vegans.

50. β-thalassaemia major

- ☐ A may present with severe anaemia between the ages of 5 and 10 years
- ☐ B commonly presents with neonatal jaundice
- ☐ C can be diagnosed antenatally by Hb electrophoresis on fetal red cells
- ☐ D is associated with atrophy of the spleen
- ☐ E should be treated with regular oral desferrioxamine to reduce iron overload

51. Fresh frozen plasma (FFP)

- ☐ A is available in the UK in 300 ml aliquots
- ☐ B is the optimal replacement fluid after major burns
- ☐ C two units should be given for every four units of SAG-M blood transfused in an operative situation
- ☐ D contains blood group antibodies
- ☐ E is approved for the urgent correction of over-anticoagulation with warfarin

52. A prolonged thrombin clotting time may occur in

- ☐ A warfarin therapy
- ☐ B prothrombin deficiency
- ☐ C disseminated intravascular coagulation (DIC)
- ☐ D dysfibrinogenaemia
- ☐ E liver disease

Answers overleaf

50. None are correct

β thalassaemia major by definition presents within the first year of life after the switch to Hb A, as production of the latter is severely impaired. Owing to normal production of embryonic and fetal haemoglobins, the diagnosis cannot be made antenatally on fetal red cell electrophoresis, but requires family DNA studies. For the same reason the neonate is not affected and jaundice does not result. Splenomegaly occurs progressively and splenectomy is usually undertaken to reduce transfusion requirements. Oral desferrioxamine is not absorbed satisfactorily, and to achieve a reduction in raised body iron consequent upon increased iron absorption and transfusion requires parenteral chelation.

51. A D E

The recently available double volume FFP may help to reduce recipients' donor exposure. After major burns 5% human albumin is the preferred replacement blood product. Rather than 'formula' replacements in cases of massive transfusion, the blood count platelet count and coagulation screen should be performed and appropriate replacement given. Blood group should be observed when giving FFP, group AB being 'universal donor' for FFP. If II VII IX X concentrate is not available then FFP provides an 'instant' correction to over-warfarinisation associated with bleeding.

52. C D E

The thrombin time tests only the conversion of fibrinogen to fibrin by the addition of thrombin to citrated plasma. It is only prolonged as a result of absent, deficient or dysfunctional fibrinogen (as in liver disease) or in the presence of inhibitors, i.e. heparin or fibrinogen degradation products (as in DIC).

53. The following are recognised to be associated with an inherited tendency to venous thrombo-embolism:

- ☐ A the lupus anticoagulant
- ☐ B abnormal structure of factor V causing resistance to degradation by activated protein C
- ☐ C factor IX deficiency
- ☐ D anti-thrombin deficiency
- ☐ E protein S deficiency

54. Heparin treatment for pulmonary embolus

- ☐ A should be commenced as a constant intravenous infusion of 40,000 u/24 hours
- ☐ B prolongs the prothrombin time (PT)
- ☐ C may cause a fall in platelet count
- ☐ D may give rise to osteomalacia
- ☐ E if 'overdosed', may be reversed by quinine suphate

55. Cold agglutinins

- ☐ A cause abnormal red cell indices when blood is processed at room temperature
- ☐ B cause rouleaux on the blood film
- ☐ C most commonly have anti-Rhesus specificity
- ☐ D are associated with lymphoproliferative disorders
- ☐ E when associated with haemolysis transfusion of packed red cells is the mainstay of treatment

Answers overleaf

53. B D E

The lupus anticoagulant does cause a tendency to thrombosis but this is an acquired disorder which, paradoxically, is usually detected by the prolongation of a coagulation test such as the APTT. Factor V Leiden is probably the most common inherited thrombophilia in which the activated Factor V is resistant to degradation by activated protein C. Previously antithrombin deficiency was the commonest. Protein S is a vitamin K dependent natural anticoagulant which is decreased by warfarin treatment so it is difficult to diagnose with confidence in patients on oral anticoagulants.

54. B C

The starting dose should be weight-related, (25 u/kg/hour); a 'standard' dose may result in over- or underdosage. Heparin's chief action is to promote anti-thrombin inactivation of thrombin and therefore to prolong the thrombin time and APTT. The APTT is normally used to control the therapy. Heparin treatment can give rise to thrombocytopenia and osteoporosis (after some months' treatment). Protamine sulphate may be used to reverse the effect of heparin in-vivo and in-vitro.

55. A D

Such 'nonsense' indices are often the first indication of the presence of cold agglutinins. They can be normalised by warming the blood to 37°c. Rouleaux are characteristic of conditions associated with a high ESR and appear similar to piles of coins gently tipped over, lying in branching chains. Cold agglutinates are haphazard collections of red cells which form when the blood on the microscope slide cools. Cold agglutinins are antibodies directed against red cell antigens which become active at low temperatures; they are usually directed against the I antigen system – 'big I' or 'little i'. Cold agglutinins are found in lymphoproliferative disorders, after *Mycoplasma* infection, glandular fever and in idiopathic cold agglutinin disease. The mainstay of treatment is to keep the patient warm.

56. Lymphocytosis

☐ A in chronic lymphocytic leukaemia (CLL) may be due to T-cell proliferation

☐ B in pertussis morphologically resembles CLL

☐ C presenting in association with skin rashes is frequently of T-cell origin

☐ D in glandular fever resembles that of CLL

☐ E is a racial variant occurring not uncommonly in people of African origin

57. In a patient with macrocytosis

☐ A the presence of target cells is in keeping with a diagnosis of liver disease

☐ B the finding of polychromasia should prompt a reticulocyte count

☐ C the finding of neutrophil hypersegmentation should prompt measurement of serum vitamin B12

☐ D the finding is normal if the patient is a neonate

☐ E the presence of a monocytosis is in keeping with a diagnosis of myeloproliferative disorder

58. In blood coagulation

☐ A the intrinsic pathway proceeds more rapidly than the extrinsic one

☐ B the intrinsic system is activated by blood coming into contact with a non-endothelialised surface e.g. subendothelium

☐ C calcium ions are required for the intrinsic, but not the extrinsic pathway to proceed

☐ D platelets play a part in the normal coagulation cascade

☐ E when the coagulation mechanisms are working normally, blood may take more than an hour to clot in a dry, plastic tube

Answers overleaf

56. A B C

Classical CLL is a lymphocyte proliferation of B cells which chiefly look small and 'mature' morphologically. Less commonly surface markers reveal a T-cell phenotype. The peripheral blood film in whooping cough may closely resemble CLL. Some chronic skin conditions (e.g. photosensitive eczema) may show circulating Sezary-like cells, and the T-cell lymphoproliferative disorders (mycosis fungoides/Sezary syndrome) frequently present to the dermatologist. In infectious mononucleosis the lymphocytes are of very different morphology, being large with plentiful cytoplasm, they resemble monocytes or sometimes blast cells. Neutropenia is a fairly frequent finding in Africans so that a 'reversed differential' (lymphocytes-neutrophils) may be found but an absolute lymphocytosis cannot be accounted for by this alone.

57. A B C D

Other causes of target cells include iron deficiency, haemoglobinopathies and after splenectomy. Polychromasia is a grey-blue tinge to the red cell staining characteristic of young red cells; if stained by the special reticulocyte stain they show the RNA network characteristic of reticulocytes. Neutrophil hypersegmentation (right shift) is found in B12 and folate deficiency. Cytopenias, monocytosis and macrocytosis are characteristic features of myelodysplastic states, not myeloproliferative disorders.

58. B D E

The 'intrinsic pathway' is more important physiologically than the extrinsic pathway and is activated by contact with non-endothelialised surfaces e.g. damaged vessel wall or prosthetic valves. It is slower than the 'extrinsic pathway' which is activated by a variety of tissue thromboplastins. Both pathways plus the 'common pathway' they lead to require calcium ions to proceed normally. The reactions involved in the intrinsic and common pathways usually take place on, and are catalysed by, platelet membrane phospholipids. Whole blood clotting time of a venous sample in a dry tube is not recommended as even the roughest guide to 'clotting ability' as it depends so much on the precise conditions e.g. temperature, trauma of venepuncture but especially on the material of the container. In plastic it may take an hour or more to clot; in glass this occurs much more quickly.

59. Oral iron treatment

- ☐ A imparts a characteristic slate grey colour to the stools
- ☐ B increases the risk of fits in patients with epilepsy
- ☐ C results in a slower haemoglobin recovery than intramuscular iron
- ☐ D may cause dose-related abdominal side effects
- ☐ E may be purchased from pharmacies without a prescription

60. The following statements are true about factor VIII:

- ☐ A it consists of two parts of approximately equal size
- ☐ B synthesis of factor VIIIc and VIII von Willebrand factor (VWF) is controlled by sex-linked (X chromosomes) genes
- ☐ C synthesis of VIIIc and VWF takes place chiefly in the liver
- ☐ D in von Willebrand's disease, there is a reduction in both VIIIc and VIII VWF
- ☐ E a factor VIIIc level of 10% (normal range 50–150%) is associated with a severe bleeding diathesis

61. in transfusion transmitted cytomegalovirus (CMV) infection

- ☐ A the risk of cytomegalovirus transmission can be reduced by leucocyte-depleting blood filters
- ☐ B more than a third of blood donors in the UK are CMV antibody positive
- ☐ C premature neonates should receive blood from CMV-negative donors
- ☐ D aciclovir is an effective treatment for CMV pneumonitis after bone marrow transplant
- ☐ E measurement of IgM CMV antibodies is the earliest method of diagnosing infection

Answers overleaf

59. A D E

The stool discolouration should not be confused with melaena. Oral iron produces the same increment in haemoglobin as parenteral iron (about 1 g/week) unless deficiency is due to malabsorption. Reducing the dose will usually improve side effects such as indigestion and constipation; if this does not work then change to another oral iron preparation. For patients who pay prescription charges it is cheaper to purchase oral iron at the chemist.

60. D

Factor VIIIc, the factor taking part in the intrinsic clotting cascade is very much smaller than the large, polymerised factor VIII VWF, which acts as a carrier molecule. VIII VWF is under autosomal genetic control (so that both sexes can suffer from von Willebrand's disease); VIIIc is sex-linked. VIII VWF is synthesised chiefly by endothelial cells, the site of VIIIc synthesis is not clear; all the other clotting factors are synthesised in the liver. The primary problem in von Willebrand's disease is reduction in the level of VIII VWF, but VIIIc is also reduced, either because its stability is reduced when it is not complexed to VIII VWF or because VIII VWF in some way controls the rate of synthesis of VIIIc. Severe haemophilia A only really occurs at an VIIIc level of 1% or less; 10% would usually be associated with a relatively mild bleeding diathesis.

61. A B C

CMV is transmitted by the white cells in the blood transfusion, so leuco-depleting is an effective prophylaxis. The supply of CMV-negative blood donors is not sufficient to ensure that all recipients at risk of serious infection can receive CMV-negative products. Ganciclovir and anti-CMV immunoglobulin are sometimes effective in post-transplant CMV pneumonitis. It is now possible to detect the viral genome in the blood of infected patients by polymerase chain reaction.

62. In a patient with paroxysmal nocturnal haemoglobinuria (PNH)

- ☐ A iron may precipitate acute haemolysis
- ☐ B aplastic anaemia is a recognised complication
- ☐ C chronic granulocytic leukaemia may supervene
- ☐ D the Hess test is commonly abnormal
- ☐ E splenomegaly is commonly present

63. In chronic myeloid (granulocytic) leukaemia (CML)

- ☐ A the predominant white cell in the blood is the neutrophil
- ☐ B absolute basophilia and eosinophilia is usual
- ☐ C the low neutrophil alkaline phosphatase (NAP) score helps distinguish this condition from neutrophilia reactive to infection
- ☐ D interferon prolongs the chronic phase of the disease
- ☐ E priapism may be a presenting symptom

64. Cryoprecipitate

- ☐ A is prepared by thawing fresh frozen plasma
- ☐ B is free of risk of hepatitis infection
- ☐ C is rich in fibrinogen
- ☐ D may reverse the platelet defect in uraemic patients
- ☐ E is of therapeutic value in haemophilia B

Answers overleaf

62. A B

Iron may indeed precipitate haemolysis and this is a not uncommon presenting feature. The mechanism may be due to increased output of complement sensitive reticulocytes following iron treatment in patients with marginal iron balance. Aplastic anaemia may supervene but there is no association with chronic granulocytic leukaemia. The Ham's acidified serum test is positive in PNH but the Hess test is not commonly abnormal unless thrombocytopenia occurs due to progressive aplasia. Splenomegaly is unusual.

63. A B C D E

The chronic leukaemias are characterised by an increased number of mature white cells in the blood, the acute leukaemias by an increased number of primitive blast cells. Basophilia is characteristic of the myeloproliferative disorders. A low NAP score is found in CML, most cases of AML and PNH. High NAP is found in infections, pregnancy and polycythaemia rubra vera. Recent MRC trials have confirmed that interferon treatment prolongs the chronic phase by a mean of about two years. Priapism, splenic infarction and stroke may be a feature of the hyperleukocytosis sometimes found in CML at presentation.

64. A C D

Cryoprecipitate is formed by thawing fresh frozen plasma from a recent donation and is rich in fibrinogen and factor VIII. It is not however free of the risk of non-A non-B hepatitis, and it contains the same degree of risk of infection with hepatitis B and HIV as other blood products, i.e. it depends on effective donor screening. It does appear to be useful in reversing the platelet defect in uraemia although the mechanism is unclear, but it is relatively deficient in factor IX and is of no therapeutic value in haemophilia B.

65. Granulocyte colony stimulating factor (G-CSF)

☐ A achieves its best physiological effect by intravenous bolus administration rather than subcutaneous injection

☐ B administration during chemotherapy improves the effectiveness of cytotoxics against carcinoma cells

☐ C can stimulate the proliferation of myeloblasts in acute myeloid leukaemia

☐ D bone pain as a recognised side-effect

☐ E increases the number of CD34 positive stem cells in the blood in normal people

66. In aplastic anaemia

☐ A a history of preceding hepatitis A is associated with a relatively benign course

☐ B immunosuppressive therapy may be effective

☐ C a leuko-erythroblastic blood picture may be present at diagnosis

☐ D ferrokinetic studies show predominant accumulation of isotope in the liver

☐ E a positive Ham's test may be present

67. A patient with a first pulmonary embolus has been on continuous i.v. heparin for five days and has received one dose of 10 mg warfarin 12 hours before blood is drawn for coagulation tests; these show an activated partial thromboplastin time (APTT) ratio of 1.7, and an international normalised prothrombin ratio (INR) of 1.8.

☐ A the heparin should be increased

☐ B the INR result shows the effect of over-heparinisation

☐ C the patient is unusually sensitive to the effect of warfarin

☐ D the aimed-for INR range in this patient is 3–4.5

☐ E the INR is the patient's prothrombin time in seconds divided by the normal control time in seconds

Answers overleaf

65. C D E

The best physiological effect is obtained by subcutaneous administration; give doses to the nearest ampoule. Administration during chemotherapy is contraindicated as stimulating granulocytic precursors into division may result in increased susceptibility of these cells to cytotoxics, enhancing haemopoietic toxicity. Some chemotherapy regimens in AML employ G-CSF prior to and during chemotherapy to stimulate leukaemic myeloblasts into division to make them more susceptible to the chemotherapy. Bone pain is most marked in patients with normal (rather than hypoplastic) bone marrow. G-CSF can be used to increase the number of stem cells in the blood prior to peripheral blood stem cell harvesting.

66. B D E

Hepatitis A may result in a serious, frequently profound aplasia with a serious outlook. At least some cases of aplastic anaemia are due to an immunological mechanism and may respond to anti-lymphocyte globulin. A leuko-erythroblastic film is not associated with aplastic anaemia but with marrow fibrosis or infiltration. An injection of Fe59 results in slow clearance of isotope from the plasma and most of the radioactivity accumulates in the liver, only a very small amount appearing in the erythrocytes. Paroxysmal nocturnal haemoglobinuria is associated with aplasia and Ham's test may be positive.

67. C

The heparin dose should be adjusted to obtain an APTT ratio of 1.5 to 2.5. This patient is correctly heparinised. Over-heparinisation can cause prolongation of the INR, which normally reflects warfarin effect. Achieving an INR of 1.8 only 12 hours after the first dose indicates increased warfarin sensitivity or abnormal liver function tests at the start of therapy; normally the effects of warfarin are not seen for 48–72 hours after starting treatment. The therapeutic INR range for DVT/PE and AF is 2–3; for recurrent thrombosis on warfarin or artificial heart valves the range is 3–4.5. The INR is the prothrombin ratio raised to the power of the sensitivity index of the thromboplastin used in the test. In simpler terms it is the prothrombin ratio multiplied by a 'fiddle factor' to bring it in line with the results of other laboratories results so that INR should be the same in any laboratory performing the test.

68. Dietary iron

- ☐ A in a normal diet amounts to about 3 mg/day
- ☐ B absorption is reduced by vitamin C
- ☐ C absorption is reduced by phosphates
- ☐ D is about 90% excreted in health
- ☐ E is absorbed in the ferric (Fe^{3+}) state

69. In a patient with polycythaemia the following support a diagnosis of primary proliferative polycythaemia (polycythaemia rubra vera):

- ☐ A increased bone marrow reticulin
- ☐ B thrombocytopenia
- ☐ C palpable spleen
- ☐ D decreased plasma volume
- ☐ E iron deficient blood film

70. Increased plasma erythropoietin occurs in

- ☐ A aplastic anaemia
- ☐ B polycythaemia rubra vera (PRV)
- ☐ C renal failure
- ☐ D massive obesity
- ☐ E hepatoma

Answers overleaf

68. C D

The normal diet contains 10–15 mg of elemental iron per day; for absorption it must be reduced to the ferrous (Fe^{2+}) state. Vitamin C is a reducing substance and therefore enhances conversion to Fe^{2+} and absorption of the element, but phosphates can form insoluble complexes with iron and impair absorption. In health, only about 10% of iron ingested is absorbed, this can increase to 30% in iron depletion.

69. A C E

The myeloproliferative disorders (polycythaemia rubra vera, essential thrombocythaemia, myelofibrosis, chronic myeloid leukaemia) share overlapping features so that increased bone marrow reticulin may be found in any of them, though it is at its most marked in myelofibrosis. In primary proliferative polycythaemia there is often an associated thrombocytosis and neutrophilia. Decreased plasma volume is a feature of the relative (pseudo) polycythaemias. Patients with primary proliferative polycythaemia frequently have an associated iron deficiency because they may run out of iron making an expanded red cells mass, and may be bleeding from associated peptic ulcer and defective platelet function.

70. A D E

Increased plasma erythropoietin levels occur 'appropriately' in aplastic anaemia in an attempt to compensate for the failure of red cell production, and in massive obesity due to the hypoxia associated with hypoventilation. Inappropriate production is thought to be the mechanism in hepatoma. In PRV and renal failure, low levels are usually found.

71. A 54-year-old man has WBC 5.4 X 10^9/l, Hb 10.4 g/dl, platelets 135 X 10^9/l. Differential count shows: neutrophils 87%, lymphocytes 6%, monocytes 3%, metamyelocytes 3%, promyelocytes 1%, nucleated red cells 3/100 white cells. The following are appropriate investigations to elucidate the cause of the abnormal blood picture:

☐ A chest X-ray

☐ B haemoglobin electrophoresis

☐ C fasting cholesterol

☐ D bone marrow aspirate

☐ E HLA typing

72. Regarding human blood groups

☐ A naturally occurring anti-A and anti-B antibodies can be IgM and IgG

☐ B most people secrete their A or B blood group antigens in saliva

☐ C the ABO type of an individual can 'change' during some illnesses e.g. acute leukaemia

☐ D group O is the commonest blood group in all racial groups

☐ E lack of certain blood group antigens protects against *Plasmodium vivax*

73. A healthy blood donor with a haemoglobin of 14 g/dl is found to have a positive direct antiglobulin (Coomb's) test. The following are appropriate investigations:

☐ A reticulocyte count

☐ B anti-nuclear factor

☐ C physical examination for enlarged lymph nodes

☐ D drug history

☐ E barium enema

Answers ove

71. A D

This man has a leucoerythroblastic anaemia: nucleated red cells and primitive white cells in the peripheral blood. Unless the patient is seriously ill this is likely to be due to bone marrow infiltration. Investigations should include a search for primary tumours that characteristically metastasise to bone (lung, thyroid, kidney, breast, prostate) as well as haematological malignancies such as myeloma.

72. A B C E

Naturally occurring anti-A and anti-B antibodies, which develop after the neonatal period, are chiefly IgM but IgG present in some group O individuals is usually detectable too. By contrast 'immune' antibodies raised after antigenic change are chiefly IgG. 80% of the population are secretors and excrete blood group antigens into saliva, sweat and tears. The A and B antigens can 'weaken' significantly during acute leukaemia sometimes to such an extent that they are no longer detectable. Group O (Rhesus 'D' positive) is the commonest group in Europeans, but there are wide racial variations, and in some groups A is commonest. Red cells that do not possess the minor blood group antigens Duffy a and b are resistant to invasion by *P. vivax*. Duffy a neg, b neg is an uncommon phenotype in Europeans, but occur in about three quarters of Negro people.

73. A B C D

Investigations need to establish whether significant haemolysis is occurring and if there is an associated auto-immune disorder. Rarely autoimmune haemolysis is associated with B-cell lymphoma. Drugs associated with a Coomb's positive haemolytic anaemia are mefenamic acid, alpha methyl dopa, high-dose benzyl penicillin.

74. A bleeding diathesis due to

- ☐ A idiopathic thrombocytopenic purpura (ITP) should be treated with platelet transfusion
- ☐ B warfarin overdose should be treated with vitamin K intravenously
- ☐ C massive blood transfusion should be treated with fresh frozen plasma (FFP) and platelet transfusion
- ☐ D haemophilia, is accompanied by a positive Hess test
- ☐ E von Willebrand's disease can be treated with desamino-D-arginine vasopressin (DDAVP)

75. The following are useful in monitoring the status of multiple myeloma on chemotherapy treatment:

- ☐ A quantitation of paraprotein level
- ☐ B white cell count
- ☐ C haemoglobin level
- ☐ D 24 hour urinary protein measurement
- ☐ E serum immunoglobulin levels

76. Vitamin B12

- ☐ A is found in meat, dairy products and green leaf vegetables
- ☐ B stores in the body are adequate for about 3 years if intake ceases
- ☐ C deficiency due to pernicious anaemia is rare in Africa and Asia
- ☐ D deficiency can impair absorption of vitamin B12 itself
- ☐ E requires replacement in patients on regular haemodialysis for renal disease

Answers overleaf

74. C E

While the bleeding disorder in ITP is due to low platelet count, transfused platelets are rapidly coated with antibody and consumed in the same way as endogenously produced ones; they are of little value and of no value at all unless given in very large quantities. Vitamin K reverses the warfarin effect too slowly to be of use if bleeding occurs. FFP should be used in this situation. Furthermore doses of more than 2mg of intravenous vitamin K render subsequent warfarin dosage control very difficult for weeks. Stored blood contains very little of the more labile clotting factors (V and VIII), and few functional platelets, so replacement with FFP and platelets is appropriate for bleeding secondary to massive blood transfusion. The Hess test is positive in situations where platelet numbers are low or where platelets are poorly functional or where there is undue vessel fragility, it is not positive in haemophilia. In mild haemophilia A and von Willebrand's disease, an intravenous bolus of DDAVP often causes a significant rise in circulating factor VIII:C and vWF:Ag and this is useful to cover bleeding episodes and minor operations.

75. A D E

The blood count will reflect the effects of chemotherapy as well as the bone marrow failure associated with marrow infiltration. The serum immunoglobulin and paraprotein levels will reflect the myeloma cell mass (except in non-secretory myeloma). The urinary protein level will also reflect the myeloma cell mass in Bence–Jones positive cases.

76. B C D

Vitamin B12 is synthesised solely by micro-organisms; the only source in the human diet is food of animal origin, (especially liver and kidney). All vegetable food is free of B12. The body stores of the vitamin (2–3 mg) are sufficient for 3–4 years, as daily requirements are very low normally, in the order of 1–3 µg. Pernicious anaemia is the commonest megaloblastic anaemia in north Europeans, but rare in Asians and Africans. Deficiency of the vitamin does cause an ileal absorptive defect, and can impair its own absorption even if the deficiency is due to dietary causes. For this reason, Schilling tests should be delayed for about 6 weeks after starting parenteral treatment. B12 is firmly protein bound, unlike folate, and so is not removed during dialysis.

INFECTIOUS DISEASES

Mark your answers with a tick (True) or a cross (False) in the box provided. Leave the box blank for 'Don't know'.

77. The following statements are correct:

- ☐ A HIV infects lymphocytes via gp41 binding to the CD4 receptor
- ☐ B normal pathogens can behave opportunistically in HIV sero-positive patients when the CD4 count falls below 400
- ☐ C HIV can directly cause renal disease
- ☐ D hypogammaglobulinaemia is an expected complication of HIV infection
- ☐ E the action of reverse transcriptase leads to the synthesis of double-stranded DNA

78. In the HIV sero-positive patient

- ☐ A diarrhoea in the immunocompromised is most often caused by protozoal infection
- ☐ B *pneumocystis carinii* is a zoonosis
- ☐ C *P.carinii* may appear as lobar consolidation on a chest radiograph
- ☐ D tuberculosis can increase the load and spread of HIV
- ☐ E central nervous system infection is a common early feature of disease

79. In the biology of prion protein (PrP)

- ☐ A the protein can be inactivated by procedures that modify nucleic acids
- ☐ B PrP is encoded on the host genome
- ☐ C PrPc (cellular) human product has the same amino acid sequence as PrPsc (scrapie)
- ☐ D it is possible, in part, to determine the risk of early or late onset of disease by studying the genotype
- ☐ E MRI and cerebrospinal fluid protein analysis are diagnostic in Creutzfeldt–Jakob disease

Answers overleaf

77. B C E

Membrane glycoproteins gp41 and gp120 are encoded on the 'env' gene and gp120 specifically binds to the CD4 receptor. The transmembrane protein gp41 is involved in the fusion of viral envelope and host cell membrane. The HIV genome is a diploid of two single-stranded RNA. A DNA provirus is inserted into the host DNA. The virus can cause direct renal toxicity. Renal drug induced toxicity is seen with amphotericin B, foscarnet and co-trimoxazole. Polyclonal activation of B cells tends to increase immunoglobulin secretion.

78. A C D

Cryptosporidia and *Microsporidia* account for 40% of infective diarrhoea; cytomegalovirus 20%, *M.avium intracellular* 10%, and *Giardia* 5%. *Pneumocystis carinii* pneumonia is not thought to arise by reactivation of latent infection but from airborne re-infection. Early in infection the chest radiograph may appear normal. Bilateral interstitial infiltrate is common but consolidation can occur. Tuberculosis can stimulate cell-mediated immunity there-by activating HIV production in infected T cells. Most CNS infection occurs late. Early, uncommon encephalopathies and presumed autoimmune disorders are reported. Classic infections include cryptococcal meningitis, cortical (grey matter) toxoplasmosis, and demyelination by JC virus (progressive multifocal leucoencephalopathy) and generally HIV encephalopathy is a late manifestation.

79. B C D

Prions are defined as 'proteinaceous infectious particles that resist inactivation by procedures which modify nucleic acids'. The normal protein PrPc is protease sensitive and no different to PrPsc in amino acid sequence. Post-translational processes modify PrPc to the infectious PrPsc. Some families with inherited prion disease have a late onset and lower risk of symptoms if heterozygous at codon 129 for methionine and valine as opposed to homozygous for either amino acid. Other amino acid substitutions are also documented both as point mutations and insertions. Biopsy is the only absolute diagnostic test in Creutzfeldt–Jakob disease. The EEG may show a characteristic 'pseudo periodic' wave activity.

80. The following vaccines are 'live-attenuated':

- ☐ A hepatitis A
- ☐ B influenza
- ☐ C pneumococcal
- ☐ D rabies
- ☐ E cholera

81. The following conditions are 'notifiable' in the United Kingdom:

- ☐ A anthrax
- ☐ B hepatitis A
- ☐ C meningococcal meningitis
- ☐ D poliomyelitis
- ☐ E tuberculosis

82. In schistosomiasis

- ☐ A eggs of *schistosoma* can be found in the urine
- ☐ B seizures and hemiplegia may occur
- ☐ C praziquantel is active against all types of schistosome
- ☐ D cor-pulmonale is a recognised complication
- ☐ E protective immunity follows infection

Answers overleaf

80. D

Except for pneumococcal vaccine which is a polysaccharide, the above false answers are all 'inactivated'. Other 'inactivated' vaccines include typhus, plague and Q fever. The BCG, measles, mumps, rubella and yellow fever vaccines are 'live-attenuated'. One of three available vaccines for typhoid is live-attenuated. At the time of writing the old rabies vaccine is live-attenuated but not the new and there are trials underway on a live attenuated vaccine for cholera.

81. A B C D E

A complete list of notifiable diseases can be obtained from your microbiology department; the following examples are notifiable: anthrax, cholera, diphtheria, Haemophilus Influenzae B meningitis, hepatitis A and B, measles, mumps, rubella, menningococcal and pneumococcal meningitis, pertussis, poliomyelitis, rabies, smallpox, tetanus, tuberculosis, typhoid and Yellow fever. Varicella (chickenpox) is notifiable in Scotland and Northern Ireland.

82. A B C D

In the normal life cycle *S.mansoni* and *S.japonicum* migrate to the mesenteric and portal veins and *S.haematobium* to the pelvic veins and vesical plexus; the first two shed eggs into the intestine and *S.haematobium* into the bladder. Ectopic ova may be found in the CNS. Praziquantel is the treatment of choice. *S.mansoni* also responds to oxamniquine and *S.haematobium* to metriphonate, however these treatments are virtually obsolete. In the presence of porto-caval shunting, *S.mansoni* and *S.japonicum* are deposited in the pulmonary vessels, leading to fibrosis and arteritis, in turn causing pulmonary hypertension. Recurrent infection in endemic areas is common. Any required immunity is, on the whole, inefficient.

83. In Rickettsial disease

- ☐ A the rash usually appears after 3 to 5 days of illness
- ☐ B focal neurological symptoms are not a feature
- ☐ C hepatic failure is common
- ☐ D early acute serology is helpful
- ☐ E chloramphenicol may be used in treatment

84. Among the sexually transmitted diseases

- ☐ A the most common cause of non specific urethritis is gonococcus
- ☐ B erythromycin is the treatment of choice for *Chlamydia*
- ☐ C untreated non-specific urethritis has a very high risk of epididymitis and urethral strictures
- ☐ D human papilloma virus types 16 and 18 are associated with cervical and anal malignancy
- ☐ E most cases of pelvic inflammatory disease (PID) are caused by *N.gonorrhoea*

85. Parvovirus B19

- ☐ A has tropism for red blood cells
- ☐ B infection usually spreads by the faeco–oral route
- ☐ C is associated with aplastic anaemia
- ☐ D increases the risk of birth defects
- ☐ E is associated with an erythematous rash

Answers overleaf

83. A E

The onset of disease is usually non-specific. Neurological signs may be absent but in severe disease confusion, ataxia, focal symptoms and seizures may occur. Jaundice is a feature in less than 10% of cases. Hepatic failure is not a recognised complication. Some rickettsial illnesses, such as scrub typhus and tick typhus have an eschar at the site of infection, whereas others such as Rocky Mountain spotted fever and epidemic typhus are not associated with eschar formation. Serological markers are of little use in the first week of illness. Oral deoxycycline is the treatment of choice but chloramphenicol can be given intravenously and during pregnancy.

84. D

The most common cause (40–50%) of non-specific (non-gonococcal) urethritis is *Chlamydia trachomatis* (type D and E). Approximately 25% of cases have no known cause. *Chlamydia* infection is best treated with tetracycline. Epididymitis and urethral strictures are uncommon. *C. trachomatis* is also commonly responsible for PID. Other organisms to consider include *Mycoplasma hominis* and *M. genitalium* and *Actinomyces israelli* (often associated with plastic intra-uterine devices).

85. A C E

The tropism for red cells is mediated through erythrocyte P antigen. Individuals who lack P antigen are immune to B19. Infection is transmitted through the respiratory route or via blood products. In the presence of chronic haemolysis and therefore reduced red cell life, B19 can cause a transient aplastic crisis by interrupting erythropoiesis over a 5 to 7 day period. Infection is otherwise usually benign though it may cause a polyarthritis. Skin rash is more commonly erythematous but may be purpuric even in the absence of thrombocytopenia. There is no evidence that B19 causes birth defects. It is associated with second trimester fetal loss and hydrops fetalis.

86. The following are commonly associated:

- ☐ A *Staph. aureus* and toxic epidermal necrolysis
- ☐ B *Staph. aureus* bacteraemia and toxic shock syndrome
- ☐ C group A strep. and erysipelas in the elderly
- ☐ D streptococcal ecthyma and rheumatic fever
- ☐ E streptococcal cellulitis and rapid onset septicaemia

87. Insect borne infections include

- ☐ A hanta virus
- ☐ B dengue
- ☐ C African trypanosomiasis
- ☐ D marburg virus
- ☐ E tularaemia

88. Amongst the complications of HIV and AIDS

- ☐ A focal skin Kaposi sarcoma responds best to intralesional alpha-interferon
- ☐ B large cell lymphomas are associated with Epstein–Barr virus (EBV)
- ☐ C opportunistic infection of peripheral nerve and muscle is uncommon
- ☐ D retinal microvascular cotton wool spots always require urgent treatment
- ☐ E abdominal pain may be due to sclerosing cholangitis

Answers overleaf

86. C

Epidermolytic toxins of *Staph. aureus* cause scalded skin syndrome. This is indistinguishable from toxic epidermal necrolysis which has a number of additional causes. However, given the number of staphylococcal infections, the association is uncommon. Toxic shock syndrome is mediated by toxins TSST1 and enterotoxins B and C; bacteraemia is rare and treatment is mainly supportive though antibiotics are required to eradicate the focal source. A rapid onset of septicaemia is an infrequent complication of streptococcal cellulitis. Group A beta-haemolytic *Strep. pyogenes* is associated with erysipelas in the elderly. Impetigo is usually superficial not affecting the dermis. Ecthyma is an ulcerating form of impetigo extending into the dermis. Both forms are associated with increased risk of glomerulonephritis.

87. B C E

Insect bites are responsible for the spread of yellow fever, malaria and dengue (mosquito), African trypanosomiasis (tse-tse fly), onchocerciasis (black fly), Leishmaniasis (sandfly), Chagas disease (reduviid bug) and tick borne *Borreliosis* and tularaemia. Contact with an infected person can lead to direct infection with Marburg and Ebola virus. Lassa fever is spread by contamination with rat urine and faeces as is hantavirus (Korean heamorrhagic fever).

88. B C E

Radiotherapy and resection are the best treatments for focal Kaposi lesions; systemic disease can be treated with vincristine, bleomycin and anthracycline. Large cell lymphomas in the immunocompromised transplant patient are nearly always associated with EBV. This is true of 50% of AIDS associated lymphomas except in the CNS which, like the transplant case, are nearly always positive for EBV. Peripheral nerve and muscle infection is uncommon. Cytomegalovirus (CMV) can cause a painful, ascending polyradiculopathy and mononeuritis multiplex. Cotton wool spots are seen in 50% of patients and are usually visual sparing and non-infectious, requiring no treatment. They may be associated with increased risk of CMV retinitis and confused with the latter. AIDS related sclerosing cholangitis is caused by several agents including cryptosporidia, microsporidia and CMV.

89. Treatment of HIV and opportunistic infection

- ☐ A zidovudine (AZT) is a proteinase inhibitor
- ☐ B ganciclovir inhibits viral DNA polymerisation
- ☐ C ganciclovir causes azoospermia
- ☐ D toxoplasmosis can be treated with clindamycin
- ☐ E clarithromycin is a suitable prophylaxis against cryptosporidia

90. The following statements are true:

- ☐ A ciprofloxacin reduces theophylline clearance
- ☐ B the folate deficiency of co-trimoxazole is attributed to the sulphonamide component
- ☐ C the azoles can induce gynaecomastia and impotence
- ☐ D quinine and quinidine can produce hyperinsulinaemia
- ☐ E cephalosporins induce haemolysis

91. Of the protozoal infections

- ☐ A pentavalent antimony compounds are the treatment of choice in trypanosomiasis
- ☐ B the Paul Bunnell test is positive in toxoplasmosis
- ☐ C amoebiasis is caused principally by *Entamoeba coli*
- ☐ D the modified Ziehl–Neelson stain will identify cryptosporidia oocysts
- ☐ E a negative stool examination excludes the diagnosis of giardiasis

Answers overleaf

89. B C D

AZT, DDI D4T, ddc and 3TC (lamivudine) are nucleoside reverse-transcriptase inhibitors. Saquinavir, ritonavir and indinavir are proteinase inhibitors. Ganciclovir competitively blocks the incorporation of deoxyguanosine triphosphate, acting as a chain terminator. Side-effects of ganciclovir include azoospermia, granulocytopenia, thrombocytopenia, anaemia and a raised serum creatinine. Toxoplasmosis should be treated with sulphdiazine and pyrimethamine, clindamycin being reserved for patients who react to sulphonamides. There is no suitable prophylaxis or treatment for cryptosporidia.

90. A C D E

The fluoroquinolones ciprofloxacin and norfloxacin increase theophylline and cyclosporin levels. This is not seen with ofloxicin. Trimethoprim inhibits human dihydrofolate reductase; the sulphonamide component of co-trimoxazole causes a leucopenia, thrombocytopenia, haemolysis in G6PD deficiency and Stevens–Johnson syndrome. Ketoconazole (not fluconazole or itraconazole) reversibly inhibits testosterone synthesis.

91. D

Visceral and cutaneous leishmaniasis can be treated with pentavalent antimony compounds. Trypanosomiasis is treated with suramin, pentamidine, melarsoprol (Gambian type) and nitrofurazone (CNS disease and Chagas' disease). Several clinical forms of toxoplasmosis occur ranging from asymptomatic lymphadenopathy, through an infectious mononucleosis like (Paul Bunnell negative) state to an acute febrile illness with maculopapular rash, organomegaly, uveitis, hepatitis and myocarditis. *Entamoeba histolytica* causes amoebiasis. *Giardia* can be excreted intermittently. Duodenal aspirate and jejunal biopsy may demonstrate the parasite.

92. In the treatment and complications of viral hepatitis

- ☐ A high faecal shedding of hepatitis A occurs in the prodromal phase
- ☐ B corticosteroids are indicated in acute disease
- ☐ C acute hepatitis B can be differentiated from chronic disease by the presence of high Hbs Ag surface antigen titres
- ☐ D chronic infection with hepatitis E increases the risk of hepatocellular carcinoma
- ☐ E chronic hepatitis is the most common outcome of acute hepatitis C infection

93. Of the atypical pneumonias

- ☐ A *Mycoplasma* are resistant to cell-wall active antibiotics
- ☐ B *Mycoplasma* induced haemolytic anaemia is associated with cold agglutinin, anti I antibody formation
- ☐ C *Mycoplasma* are Gram-positive on Gram stain smear
- ☐ D Pontiac fever is an acute pneumonic form of legionellossis
- ☐ E antibody based serological tests in legionella are highly specific

94. The following are causes of fever and pulmonary infiltrate in the immunocompromised:

- ☐ A *Chlamydia*
- ☐ B *Herpes simplex*
- ☐ C cryptococcus
- ☐ D nocardia
- ☐ E candida

Answers overleaf

92. A E

Hepatitis A faecal shedding occurs late in incubation and in the prodromal phase. Contacts should receive pooled globulin or active immunisation. Treatment of acute hepatitis is supportive; steroids are not indicated though pulsed steroids along with alpha interferon may be of benefit in chronic hepatitis B and C. The Hbs Ag antigen is present in acute and chronic hepatitis B; high titres of IgM anti HBC (core) indicates acute infection or seroconversion illness in a chronic eAg positive patient. Hepatitis E, like A, does not progress to chronic disease and is not associated with increased risk of carcinoma. Recovery is seen in 30% of hepatitis C patients. Of the remainder, 60% persist with chronic hepatitis and up to 10% may go on to develop cirrhosis and/or hepatic carcinoma.

93. A B

Mycoplasma do not have a cell wall and do not Gram stain. Pontiac fever is a short lived flu-like illness caused by legionella. It is not associated with pneumonia. It is thought to be due to inhalation of antigen from dead bacteria. Whilst serology is useful in the diagnosis of legionella (titres peaking at 4–8 weeks), they are not specific and cross react with other organisms, including E.coli and campylobacter.

94. A B C D E

Other atypicals include *Mycoplasma*, *Mycobacterium*, cytomegalovirus, aspergillosis and pneumocystis.

95. The following are features of listeriosis:

- ☐ A progressive focal neurology
- ☐ B osteomyelitis
- ☐ C cholecystitis
- ☐ D resistance to cephalosporins
- ☐ E low mortality with septicaemia

96. In *Plasmodium falciparum* malaria

- ☐ A relapse from persistent liver infection is a feature
- ☐ B parasites can synthesise pyrimidines *de novo*
- ☐ C parasite specific G6PD may be found in host red blood cells
- ☐ D primaquine is the drug of choice
- ☐ E patients rarely present later than four weeks after returning from travel

97. Features of borreliosis include

- ☐ A hepatic enlargement and tenderness
- ☐ B petechial rash
- ☐ C meningism
- ☐ D myocarditis
- ☐ E Jarisch–Herxheimer reaction

95. A B C D

Listeria monocytogenes is a non-spore-forming facultative intracellular anaerobe. Meningoencephalitis can lead to progressive neurological signs. Less common local infections include peritonitis, cholecystitis, osteomyelitis and septic arthritis. It should be treated with ampicillin and gentamicin. It is mildly sensitive to cefotaxime and resistant to other cephalosporins. Mortality rates are between 20–40% with septicaemia and meningoencephalitis despite treatment.

96. B C

Pyrimidine and G6PD synthesis can occur *de novo*; purines are exogenous. *Plasmodium vivax* and *ovate*, but not *Plasmodium falciparum*, have a persisting hepatic cycle, from which late relapse can occur. The normal incubation period is 7–14 days, but this may be affected by concomitant antimalarial therapies. Regarding Falciparum malaria, 90% of patients present within one month and 99% within six months of leaving an endogenous area.

97. A B C D E

Lyme disease is characterised by erythema chronicum migrans, fever, arthralgia, myalgia, lymphadenopathy and neurological and cardiac complications. Louse-borne (epidemic) and tick-borne (endemic) relapsing fever are associated with hepatic and splenic tenderness and enlargement, jaundice, liver failure and DIC. Tetracycline treatment of louse and tick-borne disease can produce a sometimes fatal Jarisch–Herxheimer reaction. Steroids do not prevent the Jarisch–Herxheimer reaction in louse-borne relapsing fever unlike their effect in acute syphilis; they are however useful in helping to reduce temperature and hypotension. The reaction can also be reduced by meptazinol, an opiate antagonist, and polyclonal anti-tumour necrosis factor antibody.

98. In brucellosis

- ☐ A a leucocytosis is usual in acute infection
- ☐ B the organism remains viable in dry soil
- ☐ C freezing destroys the organism
- ☐ D incidence is increasing in the United Kingdom
- ☐ E organisms can be isolated from human breast milk

99. The following statements on fungal infections are true

- ☐ A infection with *Coccidioides immitis* is usually mild or asymptomatic
- ☐ B *Aspergillus* causes paranasal granulomas
- ☐ C pneumonia is the commonest presentation of cryptococcosis
- ☐ D serology is useful in confirming blastomycosis
- ☐ E over 90% of endemic histoplasmosis infections are asymptomatic

100. In tuberculosis treatment

- ☐ A isoniazid accelerates the metabolism of anti epileptics
- ☐ B doses of oral hypoglycaemics may need to be increased during concomitant use of rifampicin
- ☐ C streptomycin can cause ocular toxicity
- ☐ D pyrazinamide may exacerbate acute gout
- ☐ E drug induced hepatitis is typically chronic and unresolving

Answers overleaf

98. B E

Brucella is a Gram-negative non-spore-forming intracellular aerobe. Typically it can be found in unpasteurized milk and soil for up to 8 weeks. The white cell count is usually normal but there may be a leucopenia and relative lymphocytosis. The UK is considered a disease free country; the incidence of the disease worldwide is increasing. Common modes of transmission are inhalation, ingestion of raw meat and untreated milk, and penetrating skin wounds. Transplacental and breast milk transfer may also occur.

99. A B E

Most infection with *C. immitis* is asymptomatic; occasionally pneumonia, arthralgia, erythema nodosum or multiforme, and meningism are reported. Most disease caused by *Aspergillus* is due to *A. fumigatus*. Paranasal granulomata are caused by *A. flavus*, and otomycosis by *A. niger*. Cryptococcal pneumonia is less common than meningitis. Blastomycosis is confirmed by culture or histology. There is cross reactivity with histoplasma antibodies.

100. B D

Isoniazid inhibits phenytoin and carbamazepine metabolism. Rifampicin is an hepatic enzyme inducer; rare side effects include thrombocytopenic purpura, haemolytic anaemia and acute renal failure. Pyrazinamide inhibits renal uric acid secretion. Ethambutol has ocular toxicity; streptomycin is ototoxic. The latter is also a weak neuromuscular blocker and causes a cutaneous hypersensitivity reaction. A transient, small enzyme rise is common with several of these agents. Hepatitis usually resolves rapidly on discontinuing therapy, but can be severe and fatal incidences have occured. Hepatotoxicity has been associated in the main with Pyrazinamide, Rifampicin and Isoniazid (in descending order of importance).

RHEUMATOLOGY: REVISION CHECKLIST

Auto-immune disease

- ☐ Rheumatoid arthritis
- ☐ SLE
- ☐ Wegener's granulomatosis

Other vasculitides

- ☐ Polymyalgia rheumatica
- ☐ Cranial arteritis
- ☐ Vasculitic disease

Other arthritides

- ☐ Reiter's syndrome
- ☐ Behçet's disease
- ☐ Ankylosing spondylitis
- ☐ Arthralgia
- ☐ Hypertrophic osteo-arthropathy

Miscellaneous

- ☐ Anti-phospholipid syndrome
- ☐ Digital gangrene
- ☐ Peri-articular calcification
- ☐ Systemic sclerosis

IMMUNOLOGY: REVISION CHECKLIST

Cellular immunity

- ☐ T lymphocytes/deficiency
- ☐ Cell-mediated immunity

Immunoglobulins/ autoimmunity

- ☐ IgA/IgE/IgG
- ☐ Autoimmune disease/ANCA
- ☐ Monoclonal gammopathy
- ☐ Tissue receptor antibodies
- ☐ Circulating immune complexes
- ☐ Hypogammaglobulinaemia
- ☐ Precipitating antibodies in diagnosis

Cytokines

- ☐ Interferon
- ☐ Tumour necrosis factor
- ☐ Leukotrines

Miscellaneous

- ☐ Angioneurotic oedema
- ☐ Complement/CH50
- ☐ Hypersensitivity reactions
- ☐ Post-splenectomy
- ☐ Transplant rejection

HAEMATOLOGY: REVISION CHECKLIST

Metabolic anaemias

- ☐ Iron deficiency/metabolism/therapy
- ☐ Folate deficiency
- ☐ Basophilia
- ☐ Macrocytosis/pernicious anaemia
- ☐ Sideroblastic anaemia
- ☐ Haem biosynthesis
- ☐ Investigation of anaemia

Haemolytic anaemia

- ☐ Haemolytic anaemia
- ☐ Sickle cell/Haemoglobinopathy
- ☐ Reticulocytosis
- ☐ Haemolytic-uraemic syndrome
- ☐ Hereditary spherocytosis
- ☐ Intravascular haemolysis

Bleeding disorders

- ☐ Haemophilia
- ☐ Thrombocytopaenia
- ☐ Bleeding time
- ☐ Fresh frozen plasma
- ☐ von Willebrand's disease

Haematological malignancy

- ☐ Hodgkin's/Non-Hodgkin's lymphoma
- ☐ Pancytopaenia/splenomegaly
- ☐ Leukaemia
- ☐ Polycythaemia

Miscellaneous

- ☐ Methaemoglobinaemia
- ☐ Thrombocytosis
- ☐ Bone infarction
- ☐ Bone marrow test
- ☐ Eosinophilia
- ☐ Hyperuricaemia and haematological disease
- ☐ Hyposplenism
- ☐ Neutropaenia

INFECTIOUS DISEASES: REVISION CHECKLIST

Viral Infections

- ☐ Hepatitis
- ☐ AIDS/HIV
- ☐ Chickenpox/measles/ mumps
- ☐ Adenovirus
- ☐ Genital herpes
- ☐ Parvovirus

Bacterial Infections

- ☐ Venereal disease
- ☐ Infectious mononucleosis
- ☐ Brucellosis
- ☐ TB/BCG
- ☐ Toxoplasmosis
- ☐ Tetanus
- ☐ Typhoid/cholera
- ☐ *Helicobacter pylori*
- ☐ Pneumonia
- ☐ *Staphylococcus*

Routes of infection

- ☐ Faecal-oral transmission
- ☐ Transmission by insect bite

Tropical and protozoal infections

- ☐ Malaria
- ☐ Tropical fever/splenomegaly
- ☐ *Pneumocystis carinii*
- ☐ Schistosomiasis

Miscellaneous

- ☐ *Chlamydia trachomatis*
- ☐ Other infections/diarrhoea
- ☐ Infections and eosinophilia
- ☐ Lyme disease
- ☐ Prion disease

RHEUMATOLOGY REVISION INDEX

Numbers refer to question numbers.

IMMUNOLOGY REVISION INDEX

Numbers refer to question numbers.

HAEMATOLOGY REVISION INDEX

Numbers refer to question numbers.

INFECTIOUS DISEASES REVISION INDEX

Numbers refer to question numbers.